Cryotherapy

I0421469

The Truth About Cryogenics: A Complete Beginner's Guide to Decrease Inflammation, Eliminate Pain, and Get Rid of Headaches

Table of Contents

Introduction

You probably have heard of cryogenics already. In 2013, cryogenics became a trending term because of a 3-year-old girl from Taiwan, whose body was frozen by her parents because she died of brain cancer, and they wanted her to get another chance at life in the future. Cryogenics has also been depicted in novels such as *80 Degrees below Zero* and *The Time Keeper*.

While cut from a similar cloth, cryotherapy is slightly different than these ideas. It involves a procedure that uses sub-zero temperatures to cure certain medical conditions. However, in this procedure, the person is still alive and would be consciously allowing his/herself to go through the therapy.

In this short and concise book, we will get into the history of cryotherapy, the science behind it, and the effects one will tend to experience. Most practically, we will also look at the pros and cons of this unique treatment method and how it compares to other similar treatments, especially when considering the short-term and long-term effects.

We are aiming to look at this topic in an unbiased light. We are not promoting the treatment of cryotherapy, per se, but we want to make sure that if someone is interested in this controversial topic, he or she can reach more informed conclusions.

We hope that you are able to learn a thing or two!

Chapter 1:

What Is Cryotherapy?

In Greek, *cryo* means cold, and *therapy* means cure. Those words brought forth cryotherapy.

Generally speaking, cryotherapy is a non-invasive therapy that makes use of whole body or localized exposure to sub-zero temperatures in order to treat certain medical conditions, such as headaches, malignant and benign tissue damage, spasms, pains, inflammation, as well as to increase cellular survival and improve a person's overall health.

This technology was originally intended to treat skin conditions, as mentioned above, but in recent years its effects in alleviating headaches have become widely celebrated.

The Process

Cryotherapy should be done in a cryotherapy facility, with the help of administrators and therapists who are experts in the subject. Mostly, you can expect a few things:

You'll have to answer a questionnaire that will determine your health problems and whether or not you are ready to undergo cryotherapy.

You'll check in and change your clothes in a locker room, if needed.

You would then enter the chamber, watch instructional videos, and then enter the cryotherapy chamber for treatment to begin.

You might go through localized cryo cardio therapy, and if you're willing, also go through localized treatment, as well as lay down in a hydro massage bed and go through post treatment stretching, if desired.

Vasoconstriction

The main goal of cryotherapy is to promote *vasoconstriction*, also known as the constriction of blood vessels. When vasoconstriction happens, the blood vessels widen, and in turn, blood loss and hemorrhage would be staunched. Moreover, tissues also begin to freeze once cell liquid, also known as cytosol, is crystalized. There are various ways in which this can work, so we'll explore these later.

Cryotherapy usually takes place in health and wellness centers, and even in European spas. Recently, it has made its way to the United States and is slowly gaining the curiosity of many.

Chapter 2:

History of Cryotherapy

As early as 2500 BC, ancient Egyptians had already learned to harness the power of "cold." Over the years, coldness had been used for amputations, which was a well-known occurrence during 1845 to 1851 by Napoleon's surgeon, Dominique Jean-Larry.

How It All Began

Possibly the first doctor who was able to explain the importance of coldness was Brighton's Dr. James Arnott. Arnott said that crushed ice in the temperature range of -18 to -24 °C was best for treating skin, cervical, and breast cancer, apart from abrasions. He also said that these temperatures worked best against neuralgia and headaches because somehow they numbed the pain and killed cells that caused pain.

It was also Dr. Arnott who started to create the first kind of Cryotherapy Apparatus, and he showed it at the 1851 Exhibition of London. The problem with this device though was that it had minimal freezing ability and couldn't anesthetize the skin the way it was supposed to. However, all was not lost because Arnott believed that at least he had been able to show the public what cryotherapy was about in principle.

The Development

In 1877, Piecet and Calleitet of Switzerland and France, respectively, began to develop this expansion system of cool gasses. Then, in 1892, the first liquefied gas vacuum flask was invented by Great Britain's James Dewar, and Germany's Von Lined helped in its commercialization not long afterwards.

In 1899, liquid air was first used in a clinical application. They used -190 °C of cold air. It was applied with the use of a brass roller device, a spray, or a swab. Again, the use of this cold air was for the treatment of skin problems, which included epithelomias, chancroid warts, herpes zoster, and erythematous. In fact, in 1907, at least fifteen patients with skin cancers had been reported to get better because of cold air treatment, mostly with the use of a spray bottle.

Innovations

In 1910, Dr. William Pusey of Chicago introduced the use of -78.5 °C solidified air, also known as solid carbon dioxide. This was the same mechanism that was used for most soda fountains at the time.

With it, Pusey was able to treat medical conditions, such as lupus vulgaris, erythematous, lichen planus, and warts. It was also during this time that dermatologists incorporated the use of freezing liquid or cold air for dermatology. Carbon dioxide was then known as the pioneering agent of the cryotherapy process.

If there was solid air, then there was also liquid air, or those in the -189.2 °C range. It was in the 1920's that this started to be used, though not many people wanted to adapt it because it was highly combustible and dangerous. However, over 1,000 people with various conditions—not just limited to skin problems—have since benefited from liquid air.

After the Second World War, -196 °C liquid nitrogen started to become available publicly.

Dr. Ray Allington then made use of it for clinical practice, mostly with the help of clinical swabs. Eventually, this was adapted for the treatment of non-neoplastic lesions, keratosis, and verrucae.

Modernization

The collaborative efforts of Arnold Lee and Irving Cooper is said to be the catalyst of modern cryotherapy. The Cryogenic Probe that they built set the standard for the rest of cryogenic systems that followed. This probe mostly worked on a pressurized tube that made use of liquid nitrogen going through three elongated tubes to reach the patient. In the middle of these tubes lied the radioactive vacuum shield that allowed for degradation of heat to provide cold air for the patients.

More innovations followed in the '60s and '70s. Apart from nitrogen, systems were created with the help of fluorinated hydrocarbons, ethyl chloride, argon, carbon dioxide, and nitrous oxide. Nitrogen sprays were also developed to help treat dermatological problems. Carcinomas also began to be treated with the help of these modernizations.

In 1968, a handheld nitrogen spray was developed with the help of an engineer named Michael Byrne, and in 1988, the trio of Toree, Kuflik, and Lubritz wrote a book regarding the dermatological effects of cryotherapy, and this has mostly been the basis of current cryotherapy processes.

Chapter 3:

The Science Behind Cryotherapy

When delving into the science behind cryotherapy, one can always trace back to the cytosol crystallization. Under extreme cold, cytosol becomes frozen, and unhealthy cells are then destroyed. When this happens, pain is often alleviated. Natural body heat is retained in this condition, so even though cryotherapy occurs, one wouldn't be able to feel the pain of said process. During this time, blood will also reach the surface and the skin becomes paler, and soon enough, arterial pressure will be regulated. This occurs within around 15 minutes or so. To put it simply, what happens is:

The ice goes straight into the cell.

The ice surrounds the exterior of the cell.

A loss of blood supply happens.

The white blood cells then are destroyed, and cells that are dirty and damaged are then driven out of one's body. After cryotherapy, the remaining damaged cells get destroyed.

Ice Pack Therapy

Remember when you were young and your parents would put an ice bag on your forehead if you had a strong fever? When you had noticeable bruises or injuries they might have placed an ice pack on those parts of the body? Well, that was a simple form of cryotherapy.

What happens in such instances is that cold air is able to decrease fiber tension, can decrease oxygen demand, enzymatic activity, and high metabolic rate. In short, vasoconstriction is achieved.

These days, there is a medical cryotherapy gun that is available to the public, in order to treat certain medical conditions. However, it's best to use for just 10 to 15 minutes or so because using it for longer can cause problems in flexibility and balance.

Ice Bath Therapy

When one undergoes ice bath therapy, his/her body goes under the state of decreased metabolic activity and blood vessel constriction. Now, under the ice bath, tissues break down and swelling is reduced. This is why ice baths are often recommended to people who go through strenuous activities, such as athletes and sportsmen.

After an ice bath, one's body will then return to a state of warmth. When the tissues have warmed up, faster blood flow occurs and body strength is recycled through cellular lymph system breakdown. Arguably, the best thing about ice bath therapy is that it not only suppresses inflammation in the body but also drives out the harmful metabolic debris that is contained in one's   muscles.

Hyperbaric Gaseous Cryotherapy

This cryotherapy technique is all about applying cold pressure on the affected area of the skin. -78 °C of cold air pressure should be used, in 400 Hz Frequency, and a pressure of 50 bars, and you can go through the sessions more than once, if you so desire. It is also said that this tends to cause the least amount of pain when compared to ice baths.

This method of cryotherapy was introduced in 1993 by Christian Cluzeau and was mostly used for:

Vasomotor problems

Muscle relaxation

Anti-inflammatory therapy

As a general painkiller

Cryogenic Chamber Therapy

In recent years, cryogenic chamber therapy has been introduced to the public as an alternative to ice packs. Basically, what happens is that the patient goes inside a cryogenic "chamber." This chamber is filled with liquid nitrogen, which makes it cold. The patient wears a bathing suit and is protected from frostbite with the help of ear and mouth protection, gloves, and socks. This then triggers analgesia, or core body therapy.

According to most patients, they have experienced feelings of recovery and have grown stronger when it comes to fighting certain diseases, such as psoriasis, itching, fibromyalgia, and rheumatism, amongst others. Apparently, the therapy also releases endorphins, which in turn makes people happier and more attentive.

However, some reports say that athletes who participated the 2011 Rugby World Cup and tried these chambers likened them to a sauna. Still, they did note that the chamber had positive effects, especially in helping them recover.

Cryosurgery

There is also a process called cryosurgery, which is used to destroy diseased or abnormal tissues. In this process, tissues are frozen at cellular levels. If you recall, cryosurgery is pretty much the pre-cursor to cryotherapy. It is also effective because even if cells are destroyed, the body does not feel weak and malignant cell growth can be prevented.

As you can see, there are various methods that can be placed under the umbrella of "cryotherapy." As a patient, it is always best to figure out which one is the right fit for you, with the help of your preferred specialist.

Chapter 4:

The Effects of Cryotherapy

What actually happens to you when you undergo cryotherapy? How does your body react to it, during and after? Let's take a look.

Fights Headaches

A study that was done in 2000 by the *Archives of Family Medicine* proved that cold temperatures could mitigate not only headaches but also the subsequent pain that was brought upon by said headaches. In fact, around 87% of the patients said that they received optimal effects from cryotherapy, and they were likely to go through it again. This is exactly the reason why it is said that cryotherapy is an incredible tool against headaches.

Decreases Metabolic Rate

When metabolic rate is reduced by ice, the need for oxygen is lessened and vasoconstriction happens the way it should. What happens next is that damaged cells are killed, but the death of healthy cells is decreased so that one doesn't suffer from other medical conditions, for which risks might be heightened by cryotherapy.

Reduced Muscle Spasms

Muscle spasms are one of the body's main responses to pain. This happens because there are muscles that surround the injury and they "think" that they have to protect the body by contracting themselves once an injury occurs. This type of reaction is called *muscle guarding*. Because ice can numb pain in the muscles, it is said to be best used against muscle spasms.

However, this does not mean that the effects of cryotherapy on muscle spasms are limited to spasms alone. Muscular imbalances and muscle overuse issues can also be reduced by cryotherapy, mainly because of the velocity of nervous and muscular systems that are affected. Some say that muscle activity is reduced because of this, though, mainly due to what cryotherapy does to muscle spindles.

Reduces Bleeding and Swelling

When it comes to decreasing inflammation, ice mainly works to constrict blood vessels. What happens here is that vasoconstriction is brought upon by the lack of blood that travels through the affected areas and throughout the whole body. Blood then returns to the area after just a couple of minutes. This phase is called a *hunting response*.

One can liken this experience to how one may feel after putting their fingers in extremely cold water or ice. Once this happens, your body then prepares to face the problem head on, and that is why pain is reduced.

Functional loss is also lessened because blood can now continually flow to the area, after ice has been applied. Pressure in the tissue is also increased because of the anti-inflammatory responses to swelling, as certain chemicals that are inside the body are tapped and released. When you get to apply ice yet again, pain is decreased even further.

Improves Sleep

Possibly one of the best things about cryotherapy is that it helps one get to sleep better. Sleep is often a problem for most busy people, so it's just right that they find something that will be able to relax their minds and help them sleep without any interruptions, while also providing numerous other benefits to their body.

Chapter 5:

Pros and Cons of Cryotherapy

Just like with any type of intentional healing process that we subject our body to, there are important pros and cons when it comes to cryotherapy.

Pros

You feel happier

Laughter is often related to a release of endorphins in one's system. Furthermore, when endorphins are released, laughter becomes more of an enjoyable experience. In a study conducted in 2006 by the *FASEB Journal,* it was documented that people with more released endorphins laughed healthier and longer than those who didn't have as much.

Pain will be relieved

The hypothalamus is the part of the brain that is responsible for releasing endorphins, helping you drive your mind away from pain. Chronic pain is then managed better once endorphins are released. This is also an effective strategy to employ after a surgery has been performed.

Exercise

Endorphins are released when one is exercising. However, when one already has enough endorphins in his or her system before even exercising, they will notice that they will also be able to exercise even better and won't feel weak or tired right away.

Pain Threshold is Increased

Other than masochists, most people do not enjoy the feeling of pain. However, life is under no obligation to make sure that one doesn't suffer from pain.

It is said that a combination of genes, gender, and stress issues could be the reason why some people have a low pain threshold. The body releases a couple of endorphins called *betas* that try to minimize the pain after an injury. Some people do not have natural amounts of this endorphin in their body though, and the result is that a person like this could resort to painkillers in order to alleviate their pain.

But, after undergoing cryotherapy, betas can be released, and when this happens the five senses will be dulled for a bit. Then, pain gets to be alleviated, and one may not experience the same episodes of migraine anymore.

Decreased Nociception

Nociception is the term given to the condition where harmful stimuli are processed in the nervous system. You see, when you slip and fall, it's not just your body that suffers—the mind does, too. This is because there are free nerve endings in your body that act as receptors, so they tell the brain that something awful happened and that you are—and should be—in pain.

The signals then travel from nerve fibers going from the spinal cord all the way to the brain. Then, autonomic responses occur, and you may start crying or screaming about the pain that you are feeling.

Pain receptors are found in the skin, body organs, and even bones and joints. This is the exact reason why you may truly feel pain from the inside, and when you have little threshold for it, it is obviously hard to deal with. When one goes through cryotherapy, these nerve endings are numbed down.

Pain Gate Theory

There is something called the *Pain Gate Theory*, a term coined by Patrick David Wall, back in 1965. Basically, this term regards the use of a non-painful agent to drive pain away. In this case, the non-painful agent is cryotherapy.

One's perception of pain is altered after he or she is subject to the non-painful agent—so the body then learns how to deal with it better, which furthers the notion that pain isn't only a physical thing.

Cons

Changes in Skin Color

After going through a cryotherapy session, the skin on most people turns to a white, pale tone, and it can even be considered "ghostly." Of course, to those not ready for this, it can be very shocking and even frightening. While this typically does not last for longer than a few hours, there have been cases in which a patient's normal skin tone did not return for a few months.

Scarring

There are also times when scars may become prevalent, especially if deep skin areas were affected by freezing. Just as too much heat can burn the skin, extremely cold conditions can do the same.

In some cases, scarring happens when cryotherapy is done for more than 10 to 15 minutes. As mentioned earlier, this isn't healthy for the skin and not practiced by reputable experts. Just like with most of the potential drawbacks of cryotherapy, this most likely will not occur if you undergo the proper protocol.

Ulcers and Blisters

When ulcers and blisters show up, it usually means that the affected areas have been infected even further, possibly because the skin is not comfortable with the extreme cold condition. You can liken this to frostbite.

If you notice blisters or ulcers on the skin, or if skin lesions stay prevalent even after the wounds have healed, this may mean that something is wrong and you have to go to a doctor as soon as possible. You should also consult with a doctor during times in which swelling or redness is present even weeks or months post-therapy. Scabs should be gone in just 1 to 3 weeks, and anything more than that needs to be addressed with the help of an expert.

Body Pain

Some people who have undergone cryotherapy have said that they experienced a substantial amount of pain in their bodies, up to three days after the therapy. Some have said that this made them feel like resting, even if they had lots of work to do, and that they didn't seem energetic at work. If you are the type who is always busy and wants something that probably won't interfere with your responsibilities, then you will need to consider this, especially for your first few therapy sessions.

Chapter 6:

Cryotherapy vs. Cryonics

Once you understand the general principles and guidelines regarding cryotherapy, it is important to also learn about cryonics in order to understand the options and main differentiators between the two.

Cryogenics can be defined as the study of how to produce and use low temperatures for healing or improving one's health. It involves cryosurgery, cryotronics, cryoelectronics, and cryoethics - the ethical implications of cryonics itself.

On Cryonics

Cryonics is the term that is used in describing the preservation of dead humans and animals at their freezing points, until the time for resuscitation occurs. Of course, there is no clarity as to when this would be, but it provides hope for friends and families.

The reason why this is done is due to the fact that chemical activity is instantly stopped once the body is submerged in very low temperatures. Because ice forms during freezing, the tissues that may cause further damage and decay to the skin are stopped and dispersed. In short, in case these people wake up in the future and get the cure they were looking for, their bodies would be extremely healthy. The formation and structure of cells are also altered in such a way that they wouldn't age like a normal human would and should.

Certain animals, such as polar bears, have the capacity to freeze some parts of their bodies so that they don't get that affected by various medical conditions, but humans have to go through cryonics because they can't naturally do this.

Low temperatures provide cell longevity, but even to this day, there is still an ongoing debate as to whether this could really work or not. As you might expect, there are also some risks to this process. Most notably, these are:

Intracellular ice could be fatal for one's cells.

Intracellular ice could be brought upon by cell mitigation, which could stress even dead cells and could bring forth a lot of overall stress to the body.

Extracellular ice formation may occur, which can cause permanent damage to cell membranes. When cell membranes are damaged, one can expect that the rest of his or her cells and tissues won't work the way they were supposed to.

High concentration of solutes may actually damage the cells.

Cryotherapy is something that can provide instant relief. The relief is noticeable and can change your experience the same day you undergo it. On the other hand, cryonics is still being tested, and as of this day, there is still not one person who has been able to wake up from the "frozen state" in those cryonic chambers.

Cryotherapy is something you can choose for yourself, while cryonics is something that other people may choose for you—or you could also do so yourself by writing about it in your will.

With cryotherapy, you have various choices. You could go for hyperbaric chambers, ice baths, ice packs, or buy air sprays for yourself. With cryonics, your body will be sitting in one of those chambers until the day for resuscitation happens.

When it comes to ethical concerns, cryonics obviously poses some interesting debates. This is because of the fact that no one knows when "the cure" for what the person is looking for will come — it could be two weeks, two hundred years, or two centuries. Would you still know the people around you? Would you know why you are there in the first place? This crazy world of technology that we live in today would be very stressful and hard to adapt to for someone frozen in the 1970s and woken up today as a full-grown adult. These are all things to consider.

Chapter 7:

The Future of Cryotherapy

Finally, let's talk about the future of Cryotherapy. For those in the industry, this is a very exciting topic. For simplicity, we will keep this brief and non-technical for the layman. If you are interested in learning more about this interesting subject, then feel free to check out the technical writings on this subject.

As there have been a lot of innovations over the past few decades when it comes to this field, one can expect that the next few decades will be spent trying to make this wonderful experience more accessible to the general population. Obviously, this is much easier said than done.

There has been one notable Cryotherapy item released in the market as of late - *CryoPen*.

CryoPen

The CryoPen is described as a linear and state-of-the-art cooling technology in the form of a pen! It's quite portable you can use it whenever you feel like it.

It has been said that what is great about this item is that there are extremely low risks in terms of side effects, mainly because you wouldn't be subject to dangerous liquids and gasses. Freeze temperatures are also said to be more precise, plus there's also the fact that you may feel more control over the process because you can apply it yourself, instead of waiting for instructions and the like.

The CryoPen is also said to reduce the risk of burns and gives the person a higher pain threshold as well. There is no need for anesthetics, and there is minimal chance of scarring. It is mostly recommended for cases of:

Lentigo

Warts

Seborrheic Keratosis

Dermatafibroma

Non-Recurrent Basal Cell

Skin Tags

Keloids

Actinic Keratosis

Molluscum

The use of the CryoPen for Podiatry and Gynecological processes is being studied as well. As you can see, this means that, in the future, Cryotherapy may not just be limited to healing inflamed spots, headaches, and pain but could also work for other medicinal purposes.

Will Cryotherapy continue to grow?

The question here really should be, are people willing to give it a chance?

There is basically nothing wrong with trying this therapy out and also nothing wrong with opting not to. Because Cryotherapy isn't a medical procedure, one can expect that many people are going to think twice about it and would probably not go through with it. However, because these are modern times that we're living in, we can also expect that people's minds are more open to new innovations, especially when it comes to the improvement of their health.

Over time, one could expect that, aside from the *CryoPen*, more innovations will come. Cryogenic experts from all over the world are surely doing their best to figure out how this field can improve human and animal life. In time, products that are portable, that are hopefully affordable, and that humans will appreciate can come to fruition.

There's also a chance that this is the end for this technology - maybe there will be no more innovations and it won't be around in years to come. But realistically speaking, this thought is quite a little too farfetched. The amount of brilliant minds working in this industry could just be too much to allow it to fail.

Conclusion

Thank you for reading this! We hope this short, concise book was able to teach you a thing or two about cryotherapy.

Now that you understand the important factors regarding cryotherapy, you can decide if you want to try it, or if you can inform your friends who ask you about it. Plus, a little addition to your knowledge doesn't hurt, right? Our world is becoming increasingly interested in the use of alternative treatment methods, in hopes to enhance the human experience on Earth.

If you've learned anything from this book, please take the time to share your thoughts by sending me a message or even posting a review to Amazon.

Thank you and good luck in your journey!